PLYOMETRIC EXERCISES WITH THE MEDICINE BALL

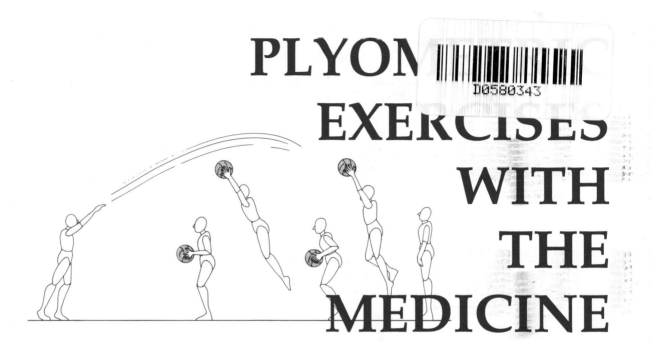

Dr. Donald Chu

Cover design by Mac Smith

Illustrations by Rie Ishikawa

Quotation on back cover by John Brant and reprinted with permission from
Outside Magazine, Mariah Publications Corp. © 1988

Library of Congress Catalog Card Number: 89-60633
International Standard Book Number: 0-931255-05-8

Printed in the United States of America

Published by Bittersweet Publishing Company
P.O. Box 1211, Livermore, California 94550

CONTENTS

Dr. Donald Chu is a Professor of Kinesiology and Physical Education at California State University, Hayward. He received his doctorate in physical therapy and physical education from Stanford University and is a certified NATA athletic trainer and a certified NSCA strength coach.

Don is currently owner and director of the Ather Sports Injury Clinic in Northern California which has pioneered the field of specialized physical therapy for sport-related injuries. The clinic also serves as a training center for Olympic bound and championship athletes.

Don has served as both assistant and head coach for the track and field program at California State University, Hayward. In 1978 he was named Far Western Conference Coach-Of-The-Year. Now he specializes in coaching high, long and triple jumpers, and has produced over 42 NCAA Division II All-Americans and 9 NCAA II National Champions. He has been represented by high jumpers in the Olympic Sports Festivals, the Olympic Trials, and the 1988 Summer Olympics.

Don has also trained national caliber ice skaters, tennis players, and members of the NFL and NBA. He currently works as a strength and conditioning consultant for the Golden State Warriors. For his involvement in improving the fitness of athletes and in the training of the general public, the Jaycees of America named him one of the ten top fitness leaders in America for 1987.

Plyometric exercise is a system of training that Don has been credited with bringing to popularity on a national level. He has traveled and lectured on the plyometric system of training in nearly every state and in several foreign countries. He serves as an associate editor for the *National Strength and Conditioning Association Journal* and the *Journal of Applied Sports Science*. He has acted as consultant to Joanie Greggains and her nationally syndicated television fitness show, "Morning Stretch."

INTRODUCTION

Optimum performance of an athlete requires two complementary abilities: skill and power. All sports from ice skating to basketball share this feature. This book describes exercises designed to develop power, particularly the speed component of power, in the upper extremities, trunk, and lower extremities. It also includes exercises specifically for wheelchair athletes.

Skill is derived from both natural abilities and learned technical expertise. The learned portion of skill takes years of training under the supervision of a qualified coach.

Similarly, power is derived from both natural abilities and developed muscle characteristics. In addition to years of muscle conditioning, power requires an integrated program to develop its two complementary components, strength and speed. While weight training develops strength, plyometrics develops the explosiveness called speed.

The aging process often brings comments like "when I was young I would have caught that pass." Slowing down or loss of power does not reflect loss of skill, and can be reversed or at least postponed by a combined weight training and plyometric exercise program similar to one used by championship athletes.

First successfully used in Eastern Europe, plyometrics is now generally accepted in the United States as a key to the training of successful championship athletes. More recently it has become a part of the general public's exercise regimen.

Plyometrics conditions the body through dynamic, resistance exercises. In its early development plyometrics was used for conditioning the lower extremities by performing jump type exercises. Now plyometrics has been adapted to improve upper extremity and trunk power by using a weighted object such as a medicine ball to create the necessary resistance.

Although it improves strength, lifting weights does not lend itself to sport-specific, speed conditioning. First, machines and free weights do not readily conform to specific sport movements. Second, speed of movement is often limited by the mechanics of machines and by the large loads used in free weights.

By using a medicine ball to create the necessary resistance for the exercises, you can experience the entire range of motion which resembles that of your sport. In other words, using the medicine ball you can tailor your exercise program to match your training needs. These sport-specific exercises are not only more efficient in developing the power you desire, they are also more interesting, more challenging, and more motivating. By having medicine balls of different weights and an occasional partner with whom to work out, you can finish a complete and specific training program in a short amount of time.

The wide variety of exercises presented in this book demonstrates the flexibility of the medicine ball in a plyometric exercise program. Using your own imagination you can continually create new exercises.

The idea behind plyometrics is simple: exploit the muscles' cycle of lengthening and shortening to increase power. Plyometric exercises start with rapid stretching of the muscle (eccentric contraction) followed by a shortening of the same muscle (concentric contraction). The goal of plyometrics is to train the nervous system to react quickly to the lengthening of the muscle by rapidly shortening the same muscle with maximum force. This process is called the *stretch-shortening cycle*.

The success of plyometric exercises is based on the utilization of the *serial elastic properties* and *stretch-reflex properties* of the muscle. Loading the muscle during rapid eccentric (lengthening) contractions increases internal muscular tension which in turn produces stronger dynamic concentric (shortening) contractions during movement. Under these loading conditions, the body is able to produce force with maximum metabolic efficiency or more powerful movements with less effort.

For example, picture a basketball player on a break away going in for a slam dunk. As the player takes his last step before going up to the basket, the one leg that is still on the floor is supporting his full body weight. This loaded leg has the responsibility of stopping the player's forward motion and changing it into an upward jumping motion toward the basket. As his last step is being taken, the muscles are undergoing an eccentric contraction (lengthening). The nerves in the leg must immediately fire and cause the muscle to concentrically contract (shorten) or the player will buckle at his knee and fall to the ground instead of going upward toward the basket.

The *amortization phase* of a plyometric exercise is the time it takes to reverse the direction of motion. If you step off a high box, then explode upward after landing on the ground, the amortization phase is the time spent on the ground. If you catch and toss a medicine ball, it is the time it takes to stop the motion of the ball and send it back in the direction from which it came. The better an athlete becomes, the shorter the amortization phase, and the greater the forces developed.

Plyometric exercises have long been used to develop power in the lower extremities by performing various jumping movements which are classified as in-depth jumps and bounds. These exercises use the body weight as the resistance force (load). To adapt plyometrics to the upper extremities and trunk, you must develop a suitable method for producing similar resistance forces.

To chose an appropriate loading system for upper extremity and trunk plyometrics, consider the differences between the upper extremities and trunk, and the lower extremities. First, the muscles of the upper extremities and trunk are smaller. Second, the ligamentous stability of the upper extremities and trunk are less. Third, the bases of movement for the upper extremities (scapulae) are more mobile than for the lower extremities (hips). Consequently, you do not need as large an external force on the upper extremities and trunk to create the ideal stretch-shortening contraction for plyometric exercises.

The medicine ball is the perfect device for imposing plyometric loads on the upper extremities and trunk. It can also be used to impose plyometric loads on the legs.

The versatility of the medicine ball is useful in developing a plyometric exercise program. You can develop a varied and sport-specific program consisting of throwing and catching movements for the upper extremities, rotational exercises for the trunk, extension exercises for the lower extremities, and finally, total body exercises.

Using a program of plyometric exercises athletes should develop a three stage program. The first stage is pre-season when the athlete often works by himself or herself and concentrates on general body conditioning. The second stage is at the beginning of the season when sport-specific conditioning begins with a partner or in a group. The third stage is during the season when the athlete maintains conditioning with sport-specific exercises. The chart on page 14 is a typical plyometric exercise program.

Each stage of the program should consist of exercises designed to benefit specific physiological systems of the athlete. An effective regimen is accomplished by both the correct choice of exercises, and the control of three variables: *intensity, duration, and recovery.*

Intensity. In weight training programs, intensity is controlled solely by the amount of weight lifted. Similarly, in a plyometric program utilizing the medicine ball, intensity can be controlled through the weight of the ball. By controlling the weight you can develop a progressive loading scheme which results in maximum speed and strength in the muscles used.

Unlike weight training, the medicine ball allows intensity to be controlled by the speed of movement. Since speed is a cornerstone in the development of power you can improve the power aspect of your training by increasing speed in the exercise movements.

Finally, the distance you throw the ball to a partner provides another method of intensity control which is not available in weight training. The farther the distance between partners, the greater the effort required to throw the ball back and forth.

Duration. Endurance comes in two forms: cardiovascular and muscular. To increase cardiovascular endurance you must raise your heart rate to 140-160 beats per minute and maintain it for 20 to 30 minutes. Circuit training is one of the most efficient methods of increasing cardiovascular endurance. By utilizing a circuit training format with the medicine ball, you can achieve fitness in both cardiovascular and muscular endurance.

The lighter load of a medicine ball, as opposed to your body weight in lower extremity plyometric jumping exercises, allows you to sustain many more efforts. Performing anywhere from 15 to 25 repetitions per station at 10 to 15 stations would not be unreasonable.

Recovery. Recovery is a key variable in determining if you are developing power or muscular endurance. Longer recovery periods (45 to 60 seconds) between sets are intended to allow you maximum recovery between efforts.

This method of training is strictly anaerobic (without oxygen) in nature and allows maximum energy to be stored within the muscles prior to single, maximum efforts (maximum power).

Shorter recovery periods (10 to 15 seconds) are intended to stress the aerobic threshold and develop muscular endurance by increasing the continuum of exercise.

Virtually no recovery between repetitions (less than two seconds) makes the exercise aerobic when you continuously exercise for 12 to 20 minutes (maximum strength and muscular endurance).

Getting a medicine ball that works for you requires some consideration. The exterior cover or shell of the medicine ball can be made of leather, rubber or polyurethane.

Although leather is the traditional material for the shell of the medicine ball, it has some drawbacks. The stitching on leather medicine balls is subject to failure. The use of leather in the outdoors is limited to dry conditions because absorption of water can be detrimental on the life span and weight of the ball.

Rubber and polyurethane medicine balls are available which remedy drawbacks of leather balls, although it is currently difficult to find a good selection.

A series of differently weighted medicine balls is desirable. A choice of balls allows you to increase the loads progressively and to change the loads in order to provide changing stimuli to the muscles. It is also necessary to have lighter medicine balls for one-arm exercises, and heavier ones for two-arm exercises.

TYPICAL PLYOMETRIC EXERCISE PROGRAM

	Pre-Season	Beginning-Of-Season	In-Season
	General Body Conditioning	Sport-Specific Conditioning	Sport-Specific Maintenance Conditioning
	With or Without Partner	With and Without Partner	With and Without Partner
Intensity (pounds)	2-9	2-15	4-15
Frequency (times/week)	2-5	2-3	1-2
Number of Exercises	5-16	10-12	6-10
Number of Repetitions	10-15	15-20	8-10
Number of Sets	1-3	1-4	1-3

Progression:

1. Increase repetitions
2. Increase sets
3. Shift from tosses to throws
4. Emphasize different body areas on different days while maintaining the total amount of work done. For example, on Monday emphasize arms, on Wednesday emphasize trunk, and on Friday emphasize legs.

CLASSIFICATION OF EXERCISES

The plyometric exercises have been divided into categories. Many exercises are clearly designed to develop a specific part of the body: arms, trunk, and legs. The sections dedicated to these areas are further subdivided into individual exercises and partner exercises. Keep in mind that some partner exercises can be done alone by using a wall to return the ball.

Because of the direct relationship between throwing and many sports, there is an entire section specifically on passing exercises. Passing refers to both tosses and throws. *Tosses* are defined as short distance passes in which the ball is passed from a position below 90 degrees of shoulder flexion. *Throws* are defined as long distance passes in which the ball is passed from a position above 90 degrees of shoulder flexion.

Other exercises are not designed to develop a specific part of the body and are categorized as general body exercises. This large category is further divided into sections which emphasize the arms, trunk, legs, and total body workout. Be aware that the classification into emphasis groups is not an exact process.

Finally, a separate section is dedicated to exercises designed specifically for wheelchair athletes.

The description of each exercise is followed by a list of several sports for which the exercise is sport-specific. No attempt has been made to make the lists complete. The lists are presented to help you see how the exercises relate to sports.

Arm Exercises
for
Individuals

Tricep Press. Stand in a stable position with your feet shoulder width apart and hold the ball behind your head with your elbows at ear level. Keeping your elbows steady, lift the ball up over your head to full arm extension and then lower it back to the starting position. *Basketball, volleyball, aerobics.*

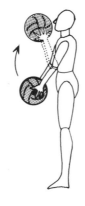

Bicep Curl. Stand in a stable position with your feet shoulder width apart and hold the ball in front of your thighs at full arm extension. Keeping your back straight, lift the ball upward to face level, and then lower it back to the starting position. *Volleyball, aerobics, bowling.*

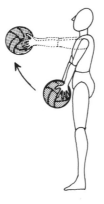

Shoulder Flexion. Stand in a stable position with your feet shoulder width apart and hold the ball in front of your thighs at full arm extension. Lift the ball upward to shoulder level while keeping your arms and back straight. *Volleyball, basketball, bowling.*

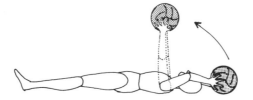

Pullover. Lie flat on your back with the ball over your head. While keeping your arms straight, lift the ball up over your body. When lowering the ball back to the starting position keep your lower back flat against the floor. *Track & field, soccer, basketball.*

Giant Circles

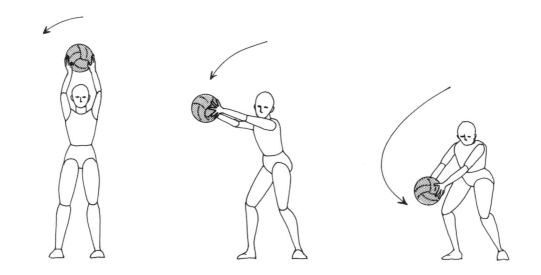

Giant Circles. Stand in a stable position with your knees bent slightly and hold the ball above your head at full arm extension. To complete a circle lower the ball down along one side of your body, sweep the ball in front of your knees, and lift the ball along the other side of your body. At all times keep your back and arms straight, and only lower your body by bending at your knees. *Track & field, aerobics, ice skating*.

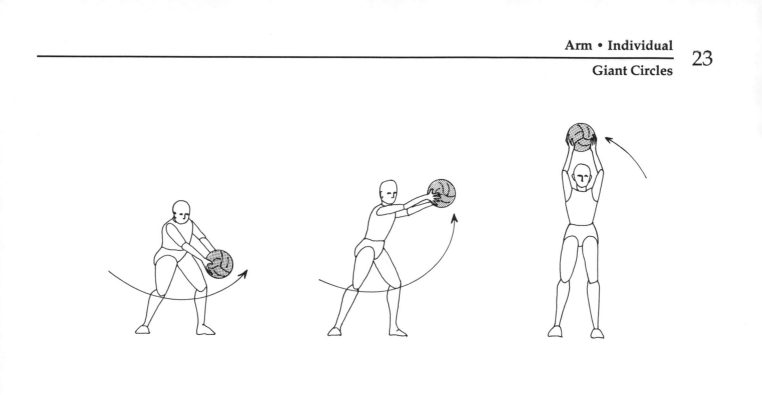

Arm Exercises
for
Partners

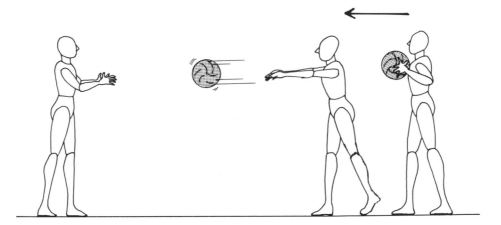

Chest Pass. Stand facing your partner approximately ten feet away and hold the ball in front of your chest with your elbows back and out. Snap the ball off your chest to your partner while stepping forward into the motion. The back of your hands should come together when releasing the ball. *Basketball, football, volleyball.*

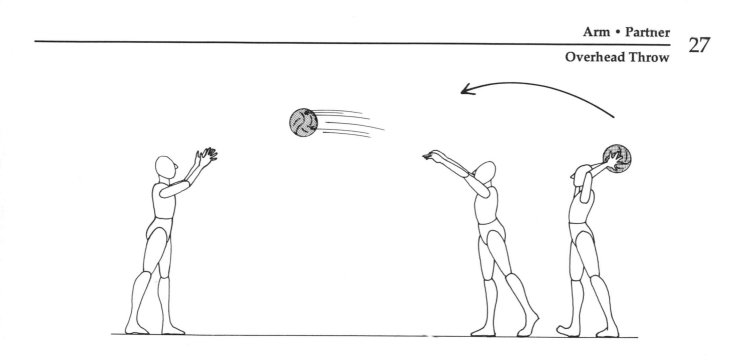

Overhead Throw. Stand facing your partner approximately ten feet away and hold the ball behind your head with arms extended. Throw the ball over your head to your partner while stepping forward into the motion. *Soccer, basketball, track & field.*

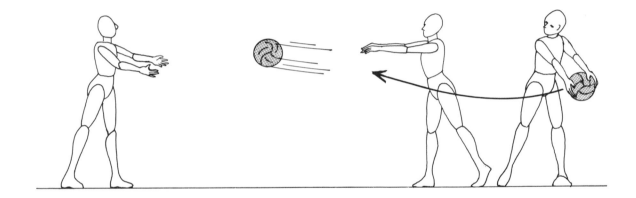

Lateral Throw. At a distance of approximately ten feet, stand side-by-side with your partner. Starting with the ball at hip level, swing it across your body with arms extended and release it at shoulder height toward your partner. When catching, turn your shoulders and head in the direction the ball is traveling to achieve full rotation. *Track & field, tennis, baseball.*

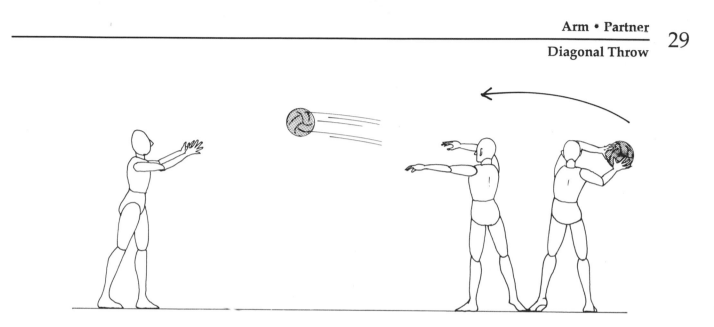

Diagonal Throw. Stand facing the side relative to your partner's position with your foot closest to your partner pointed at him. Starting with the ball at shoulder level, throw it over your head to your partner while keeping your arms extended and allowing your upper body to rotate. *Tennis, track & field, baseball.*

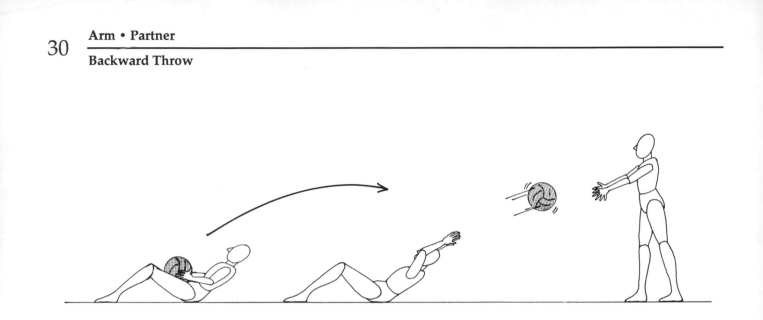

Backward Throw. Sit with your back at a 45 degree angle to the floor and hold the ball so it rests on your thighs. Your partner should stand behind you at a distance of approximately ten feet and face in the same direction. Throw the ball up and back over your head to your partner while keeping your arms extended. *Track & field, soccer, crew.*

Trunk Exercises
for
Individuals

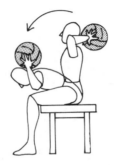

Seated Forward Bend. Sit on the edge of a bench and hold the ball behind your head with your elbows out to the side. Keeping your head back and back straight, bend from the waist forward until your chest touches your thighs. Then return to the starting position. *Ice skating, tennis, crew.*

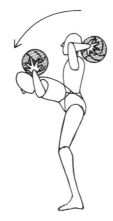

Good Morning. Stand in a stable position with your feet shoulder width apart and hold the ball behind your head with your elbows out to the side. Bend 70 to 90 degrees forward from your hips while keeping your back straight. It is important to have your knees bent slightly. *Track & field, football, baseball.*

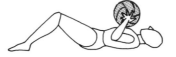

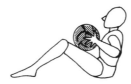

Sit-Up. Lie on your back, knees bent, and hold the ball on your chest. Lift your back and head as one unit until the ball touches your thighs. *Aerobics, ice skating, volleyball.*

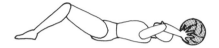

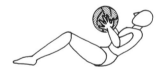

Pullover with Sit-Up. Lie on your back, knees bent, and hold the ball over your head at full arm extension. Bring the ball over your head to your chest while raising your trunk 45 degrees. Lower to the starting position in one fluid motion with the ball and your head touching the floor at the same time. *Tennis, soccer, basketball.*

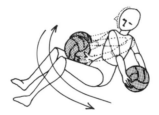

Twist. Sit with your back at a 45 degree angle to the floor, knees bent and together, and feet apart for balance. While holding the ball in front of you at full arm extension, twist your upper body and move the ball from side to side. *Tennis, football, baseball.*

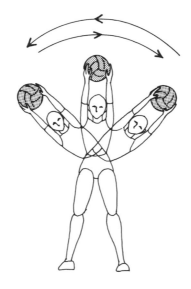

Lateral Bend. Stand in a stable position with your feet shoulder width apart and hold the ball above your head at full arm extension. Bend side-to-side from your waist while keeping your back and arms straight. Make sure that your knees are *not* locked. *Aerobics, basketball, track & field.*

Trunk Exercises
for
Partners

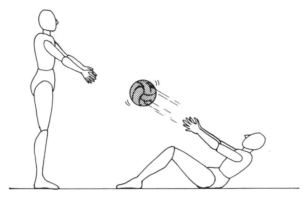

Pass Back from Sit-Up Position. Sit with your back at a 45 degree angle to the floor and hold the ball in front of your chest. Your partner can stand on your feet or move back five feet. Pass the ball back and forth. You should not move from the 45 degree angle during the exercise. *Football, track & field, volleyball.*

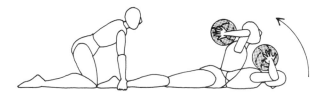

Back Arch. Lay on your stomach holding the ball behind your head while your partner holds your feet. Arch your trunk upward and hold this position for a count of five before lowering back to the starting position. *Tennis, baseball, basketball.*

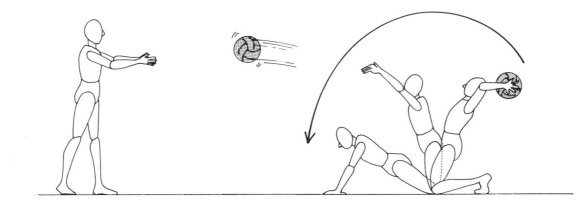

Kneeling Throw. Kneel and hold the ball behind your head with arms extended while facing your partner approximately ten feet away. Throw the ball to your partner while keeping your body straight and catch your body in a push-up position after releasing the ball. *Football, track & field, tennis, soccer.*

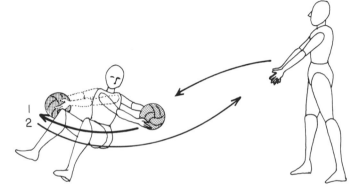

Lateral Toss. Sit with your knees bent, feet apart, and back at a 45 degree angle to the floor, and hold the ball with arms extended. Your partner should stand to the side and behind you. Rotate your arms and trunk from side-to-side and then toss the ball to your partner. A modified version of this exercise is obtained by adding more rotations of your trunk before tossing the ball. *Tennis, baseball, track & field.*

Trunk Twist with Resistance

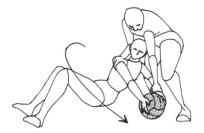

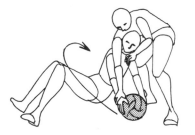

Trunk Twist with Resistance. Sit with your knees bent, feet apart, and back at a 45 degree angle to the floor, and hold the ball in front of yourself at full arm extension. Twist your upper body and move the ball from side-to-side while your partner creates work resistance by holding your shoulder and arm as shown. *Tennis, track & field, baseball.*

Leg Exercises
for
Individuals

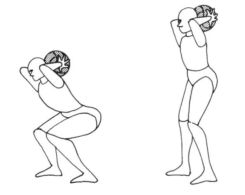

Squat. Stand in a stable position with your feet shoulder width apart and hold the ball behind your head. Lower your upper body by pushing your buttocks backward, arching your back, and keeping your head and shoulders up. The weight of your body should be back so your knees do not go out in front of your feet. *Football, volleyball, weight lifting.*

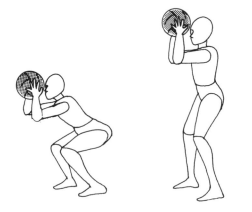

Front Squat. Stand in a stable position with your feet shoulder width apart and hold the ball in front of you at eye level. Lower your upper body by pushing your buttocks backward, arching your back, and keeping your head and shoulders up. The weight of your body should be back so your knees do not go out in front of your feet. *Football, basketball, wrestling.*

Leg • Individual

Overhead Squat

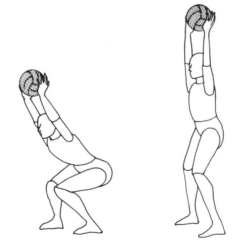

Overhead Squat. Stand in a stable position with your feet shoulder width apart and hold the ball above your head at full arm extension. Lower your upper body by pushing your buttocks backward, arching your back, and keeping your head and arms up. The weight of your body should be back so your knees do not go out in front of your feet. *Basketball, weight lifting, ice skating.*

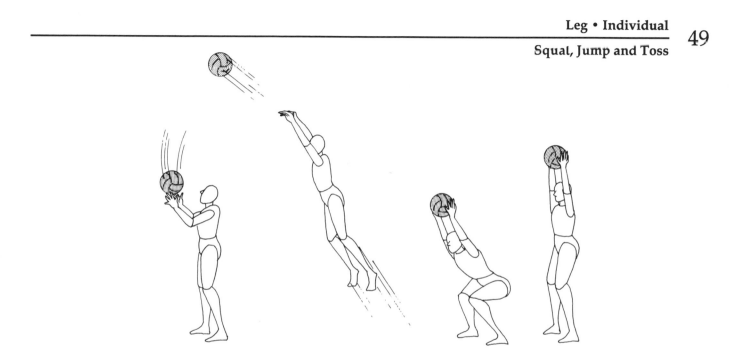

Squat, Jump and Toss. As you do an overhead squat, explode upward from the down position. While coming off the ground you can toss the ball in any direction, or throw it straight up and catch it as your body prepares for the next squat. *Basketball, volleyball, ice skating.*

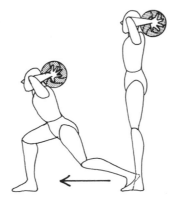

Lunge Squat. Stand with the ball held behind your head with your elbows at ear level. Step as far forward as possible and lower your body onto the forward leg. When you are stretched fully, your upper body should be perpendicular to your front thigh and your back knee should be lower than your front knee. Do not let your front knee bend past 90 degrees or let your upper body lean forward. Push back off your front foot to return to the starting position. *Track & field, ice skating, gymnastics.*

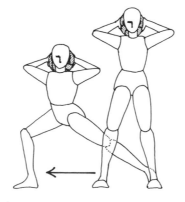

Side Squat. Stand with your feet a little more than shoulder width apart and hold the ball behind your head. Step out to one side with your foot pointed in that direction. Your step is not far enough if your knee extends past your toes. Keep your upper body perpendicular to the floor and bend your knee to 90 degrees before pushing back to the starting position. *Aerobics, gymnastics, tennis.*

Leg Exercises
for
Partners

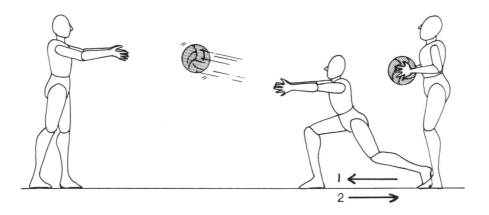

Lunge Squat with Toss. Stand facing your partner approximately 15 feet away and hold the ball at your chest. Step forward as far as possible and lower your body onto your forward leg. As you lunge forward pass the ball to your partner and then push off your front foot to return to a standing position. Your partner then lunges forward and repeats the toss. *Fencing, ice skating, gymnastics.*

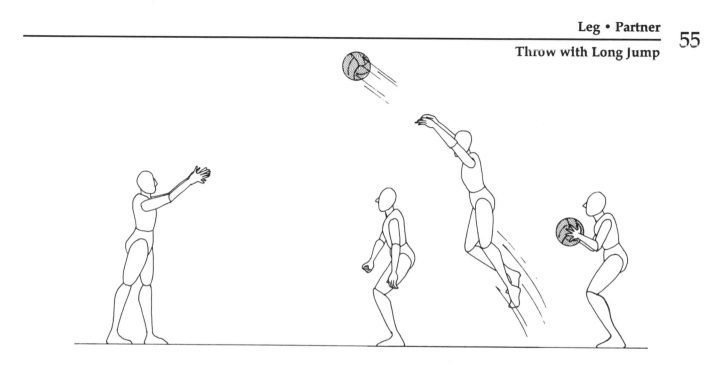

Throw with Long Jump. Stand facing your partner 15 to 20 feet away and hold the ball at chest height. As you do a quarter squat, explode upward and pass the ball to your partner. While throwing the ball, jump as far forward as possible. *Basketball, volleyball, track & field.*

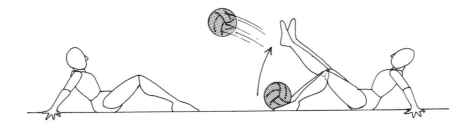

Kick Toss. At a distance of approximately ten feet, both you and your partner sit facing each other with your backs at a 45 degree angle to the floor. Place both your hands behind and to the side for support. Place the ball between your feet and toss it to your partner who in turn tosses it back. *Soccer, tennis, track & field.*

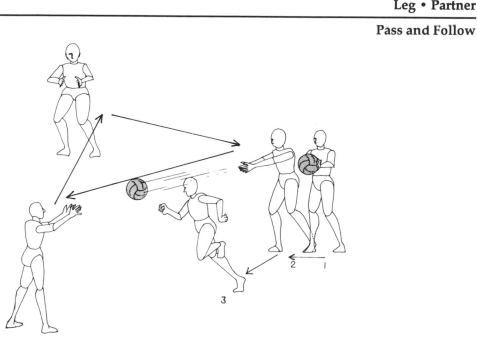

Pass and Follow. This exercise is for a group of four or more players. Three players stand at the points of a triangle 10 to 15 feet apart and additional players stand behind the front three. Starting in a corner with at least two players, pass the ball to the next corner and run to the end of the line to which you passed the ball. The pass and run is repeated thereby creating a continuous motion of passing and running. *Basketball, football, track & field.*

Passing Exercises

Supine Chest Toss

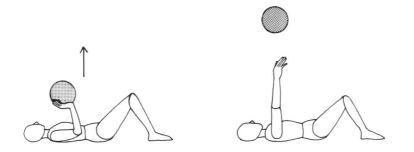

Supine Chest Toss. Lie on your back with your knees bent and rest the ball in your hands above your chest. Push the ball upward off your hands explosively. The ball should go upward in a straight line so that you can catch it without moving. *Track & field, aerobics, volleyball.*

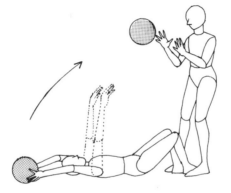

Pullover Pass. Lie on your back with your knees bent and hold the ball over your head. Your partner stands at your feet and you pass the ball to him or her while keeping your arms extended. Your partner can back up to add distance to the pass. *Soccer, tennis, track & field.*

Kneeling Chest Pass

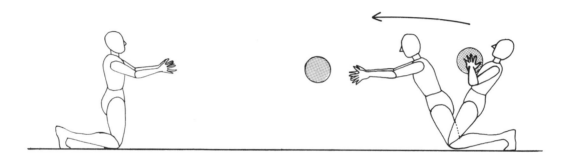

Kneeling Chest Pass. Kneel facing your partner approximately ten feet away and hold the ball in front of your chest. Forcefully rock forward while pushing the ball off your chest to your partner. Keep your stomach and buttocks tucked in, and your body straight. *Basketball, volleyball, baseball.*

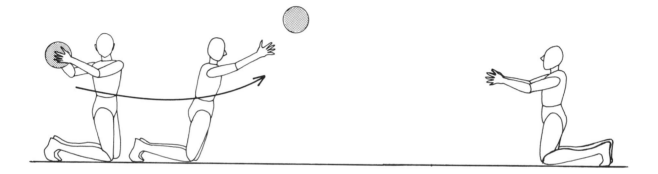

Kneeling Side Throw. Kneel facing your partner approximately ten feet away and hold the ball to one side and back behind your shoulder. Twist your upper body and arms at the same time and throw the ball forward to your partner. *Tennis, baseball, racquetball.*

One Arm Overhead Throw

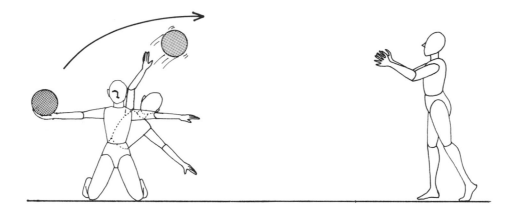

One Arm Overhead Throw. Kneel with your knees apart for balance and arms out to the side while holding the ball in one hand. Lean to your side opposite the ball while throwing the ball up and over your head to your partner. *Volleyball, baseball, track & field.*

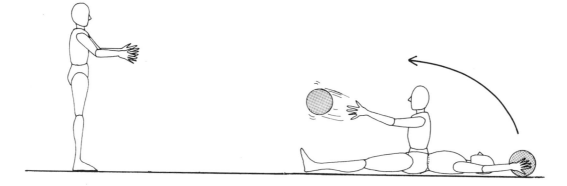

Pullover Toss. Lie flat on the floor with the ball over your head at full arm extension. While pulling the ball over your head, sit up and toss the ball to your partner standing approximately ten feet away. When your partner returns the ball, catch it and reverse your tossing movement. *Basketball, soccer, tennis.*

Backward Throw

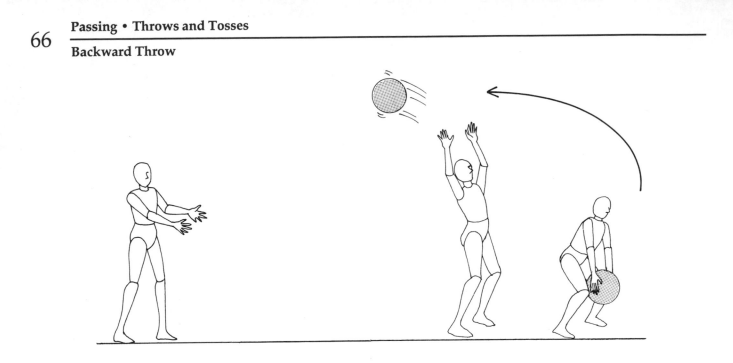

Backward Throw. Stand approximately ten feet in front of your partner and face in the same direction. Hold the ball in front of yourself, bend forward, and then toss it up and over your head to your partner. Be careful to bend your knees, bend from your hips, and keep your back straight through the motion. *Track & Field, football, basketball.*

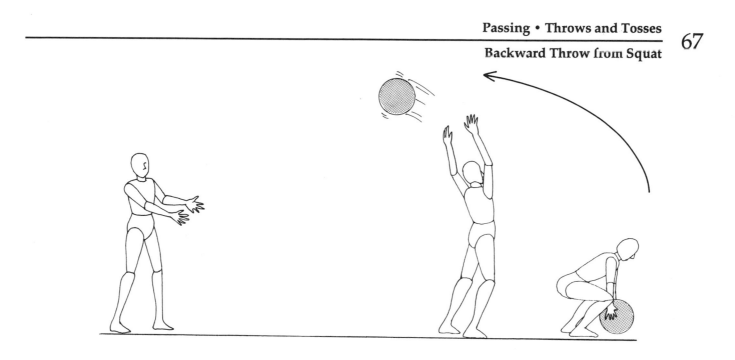

Backward Throw from Squat. In a squat position hold the ball close to the ground. Come straight up from the squat position and throw the ball up and back over your head to your partner standing approximately ten feet away. Lift your body straight up from the squat position and keep your back straight. *Track & field, football, gymnastics.*

Kneeling Backward Pass

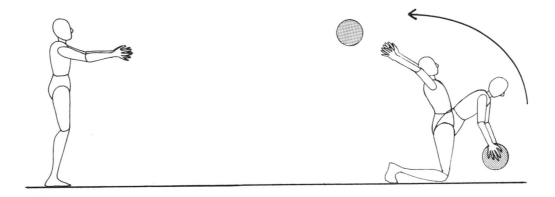

Kneeling Backward Pass. With your partner approximately ten feet behind you and facing in the same direction, kneel while holding the ball at thigh level. Lean your upper body forward, and then throw the ball up and back over your head to your partner while keeping your back straight and arms extended. *Track & field, tennis, crew.*

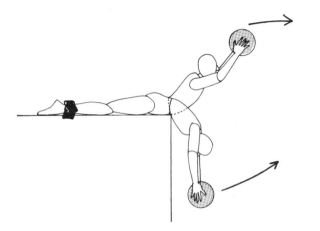

Back Hyper with Pass. Lie with your upper body hanging off the end of a table and your partner standing approximately ten feet in front of you. While you do a back hyper-extension, your partner passes the ball to you and you pass it back. The catches and passes can be done in two different ways. You can rise up to catch the ball at your highest point and then pass the ball while coming forward and down. Or you can catch the ball at your lowest point and then pass it while coming up. This exercise is easiest to do with a third partner or some object holding your ankles down. *Tennis, track & field, football.*

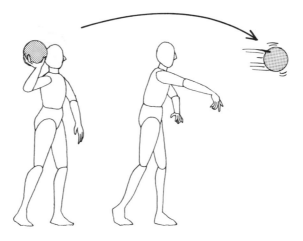

One Arm Throw. Hold the ball in one hand at ear level with your elbow at 90 degrees to your side. Step out and throw the ball to your partner. You can execute the throw by allowing your arm to fully extend, or by keeping your elbow fixed at 90 degrees and rotating your arm at the shoulder. *Volleyball, baseball, track & field.*

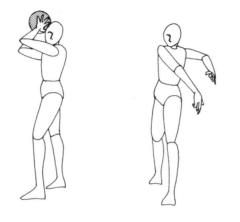

Across the Body Throw. Stand with one foot in front of the other and hold the ball with two hands back to one side. Stepping out with the forward foot, throw the ball across your body to your partner standing approximately ten feet away. Allow your upper body to twist while making the throw. *Baseball, tennis, racquetball.*

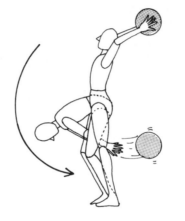

Over and Through the Legs. Standing with your feet apart, hold the ball above and slightly behind your head at full arm extension. Swing the ball over your head, down through your legs, and throw it to your partner. While making the swing downward, let your knees bend and your hips lower in order to keep your back straight. *Soccer, football, tennis.*

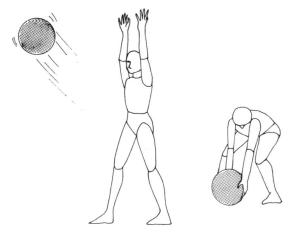

Underhand Throw. In a squat position hold the ball close to the ground. From the squat position come straight up and throw the ball up and outward to your partner standing approximately ten feet away. Lift your body straight up from the squat position and keep your back straight. *Baseball, volleyball, football.*

Pass On the Go

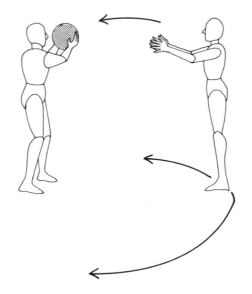

Pass On the Go. Stand facing your partner approximately ten feet away. Pass the ball to your partner while he shuffles from side-to-side a distance of 15 to 20 feet. He passes the ball back to you as he continues to move and the passing is repeated. *Basketball, volleyball, tennis.*

General Body Exercises with emphasis on Upper Extremities

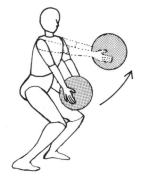

Front Raise. Stand in a stable position with your feet shoulder width apart and hold the ball at thigh level with arms fully extended. Lower your body to a quarter squat by pushing your buttocks backward, arching your back, and keeping your head and shoulders up. At the same time lift the ball up to shoulder level. Then return to your starting position. *Aerobics, gymnastics, ice skating.*

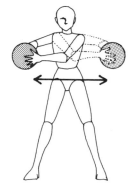

Shoulder Twist. Stand in a stable position with your feet slightly more than shoulder width apart and hold the ball at chest level with your elbows bent and pointed outward. Move the ball in a straight line across your body and past your shoulders. Do not rotate your upper body. *Baseball, ice skating, track & field.*

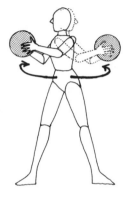

Standing Twist. Stand in a stable position with your feet shoulder width apart and your feet turned slightly outward. Hold the ball at chest level with elbows bent and pointed outward. Rotate your upper body from side-to-side while keeping the ball in front of your chest. *Tennis, baseball, racquetball.*

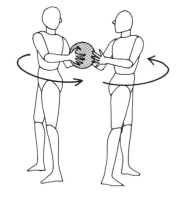

Partner Twist. Stand with your partner back-to-back and pass the ball around in a circle. The distance between you and your partner can be increased to require more twisting of the upper body before the ball is handed off. *Tennis, baseball, track & field.*

Lateral Bend

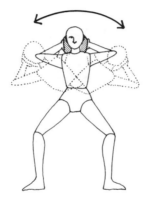

Lateral Bend. Stand in a stable position with your feet more than shoulder width apart and knees slightly bent. Hold the ball behind your head with your elbows at 90 degrees to your body. Bend at your waist from side-to-side while keeping your back straight. *Aerobics, gymnastics, bowling.*

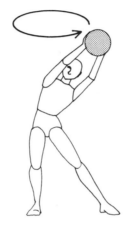

Circles. Stand in a stable position with your feet more than shoulder width apart. Hold the ball above your head at full arm extension, and move the ball and your upper body in big circles. At all times keep your heels on the floor and maintain your balance. *Soccer, aerobics, gymnastics.*

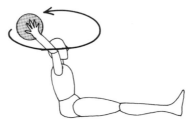

Seated Circles. Sit on the floor with your legs extended in front of your body and apart for balance. Hold the ball above your head at full arm extension and move the ball in as large of circles as possible without losing balance. *Tennis, volleyball, ice skating.*

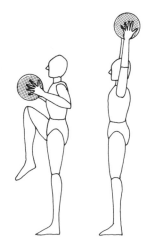

Knee Up. Stand in a stable position with your feet shoulder width apart and hold the ball above your head at full arm extension. While lifting one knee upward, bring the ball down to meet it while maintaining your balance. Return to your starting position and repeat with your other knee. *Track & field, aerobics, gymnastics.*

Hurdler Extension

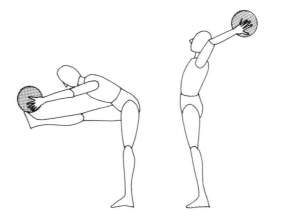

Hurdler Extension. Stand in a stable position with your feet shoulder width apart and hold the ball up and back behind the head at full arm extension. While bringing the ball forward and down, simultaneously lift one leg out straight until your foot meets the ball at waist level. Be careful to maintain your balance. *Track & field, soccer, ice skating.*

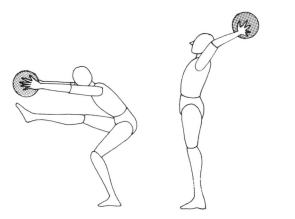

Hurdler Extension II. Do the hurdler extension as previously described, but once your foot and ball meet, lower your body down on your balance foot to a quarter squat. *Track & field, gymnastics, ice skating.*

General Body Exercises with emphasis on Trunk

Straight Arm Sit-Up

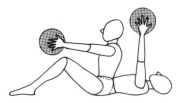

Straight Arm Sit-Up. Lie on your back with knees bent, and hold the ball above your body at full arm extension. Lift your back upward until the ball comes over the top of your knees and then return to the starting position. *Aerobics, gymnastics, basketball.*

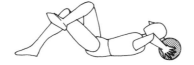

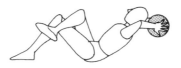

Crossed Leg Sit-Up. Lie on your back with one leg bent and the ankle of the other leg across the bent leg. Hold the ball behind your head, then lift your upper body and ball upward as a unit to a 45 degree angle to the floor. *Aerobics, tennis, track & field.*

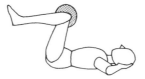

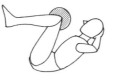

Sit-Up Crunch. Lie on your back with your knees up and legs bent at a 90 degree angle. Hold the ball by squeezing it between your knees. Place your hands behind your head and lift your shoulders up from the floor. Before lifting your shoulders, bend your head toward your chest in order to keep from jerking your head and neck. *Aerobics, gymnastics, ice skating.*

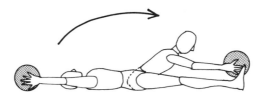

Overhead to Feet. Lie flat on your back with the ball over your head at full arm extension. Bend at your hips and bring your body and ball up and over until the ball touches your feet. *Track & field, football, soccer.*

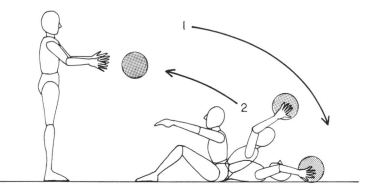

Sit-Up Toss. Sit on the floor, knees bent, and arms in front of you at full arm extension ready to catch a toss from your partner approximately ten feet away. When you catch the ball allow it to carry your arms backward and over your head. When the ball is above your head, lower your trunk to the floor while keeping your arms extended. Return the ball to your partner by reversing the motion. *Track & field, soccer, basketball*

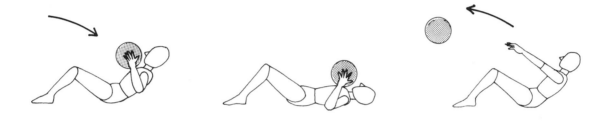

Sit-Up Toss Variation. Sit on the floor, knees bent, and arms in front of your chest ready to catch a toss from your partner standing approximately ten feet away. As you catch the ball slowly lower your trunk to the floor. Do not let the ball knock you to the floor. Return the ball to your partner by reversing the motion and tossing the ball as your trunk rises. *Volleyball, gymnastics, track & field.*

Sit-Up Roll

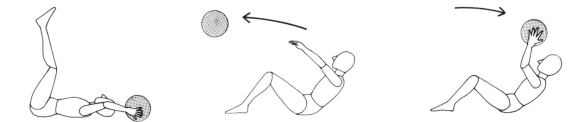

Sit-Up Roll. Lie on your back, legs up in the air, and hold the ball over your head at full arm extension. While raising your trunk, bring the ball over your head, lower and bend your legs, and toss the ball to your partner standing approximately twenty feet away. Your partner tosses the ball back to you as you go backward toward the floor and your legs go up. *Soccer, tennis, track & field.*

Seated Backward Toss. Sit holding the ball outstretched over your straight legs while your partner stands behind you approximately ten feet away facing in the same direction. Raise your upper body, arms, and ball as a unit and toss the ball up and back over your head to your partner while keeping your arms extended and back straight. *Ice skating, track & field, football.*

Hip Rotation

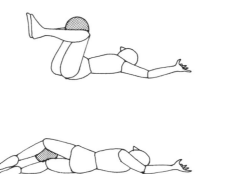

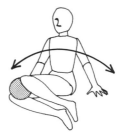

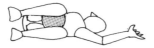

Hip Rotation. Lie on your back with your knees up at 90 degrees and hold the ball by squeezing it between your knees. Extend your arms out to the sides for balance. While rotating your hips from left to right, allow your knees to lightly touch the floor on each side. A variation of this exercise is obtained by sitting with your back at a 45 degree angle to the floor while you rotate your hips. *Aerobics, baseball, gymnastics.*

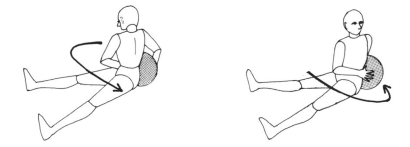

Trunk Rotation. Sit with your legs straight on the floor, legs spread for balance and the ball behind your back. Rotate to the right, pick up the ball, bring it around the front of your body to your left side, and place it behind your back thereby completing a circle around your body. *Baseball, basketball, golf.*

Trunk Exercise with Resistance

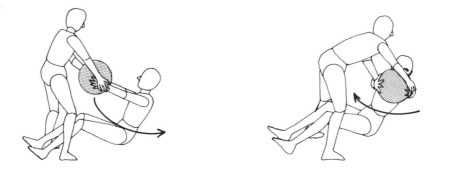

Trunk Exercise with Resistance. Sit with your back at a 45 degree angle to the floor, knees bent and together, and feet apart for balance. While holding the ball in front of you at full arm extension, twist your upper body and move the ball from side-to-side. Your partner stands in front of you, holds the ball, and resists your efforts to move the ball. *Track & field, baseball, golf.*

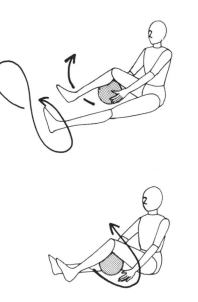

Over-Under. Sit on the floor with your legs straight in front of you. Lift your right leg and pass the ball under it from the inside out. Then pass it over the top of your right leg and under the left leg from the inside out, and over the top of your left leg. The ball makes a figure eight around your legs. *Basketball, volleyball, aerobics.*

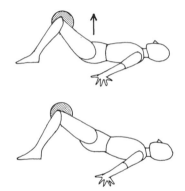

Pelvic Thrust. Lie on your back, knees bent, arms out to your side for balance, and hold the ball by squeezing it between your knees. Lift your buttocks off the floor while squeezing your buttock muscles. Either hold the up position for a count of five or do five one-inch bounces while in this position. *Aerobics, track & field, tennis.*

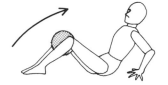

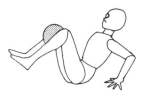

Hip Crunch. Sit with your back at a 45 degree angle to the floor, brace your yourself with your hands behind your hips, and hold the ball by squeezing it between your knees. Lift your feet off the floor and draw your knees toward your chest. You can also be do this exercise off the end of a bench so that you can move the ball through a longer range of motion. *Track & field, gymnastics, ice skating.*

Backward Sit-Up

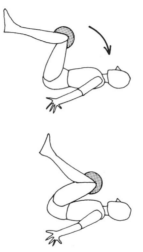

Backward Sit-Up. Lie on your back with your knees and hips bent at 90 degrees. Squeeze the ball between your knees and draw it toward your chest. Do this exercise slowly without rocking for momentum. *Aerobics, gymnastics, golf.*

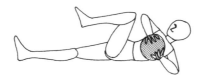

Supine Knee to Elbow. Lie flat on the floor with the ball held above your chest. Rotate your right elbow up and over your body while simultaneously lifting your left knee until they meet. Return to the starting position and rotate to the other side. This can be done quickly to simulate cycling. *Aerobics, tennis, cycling.*

General Body Exercises with emphasis on Lower Extremities

Front Toss

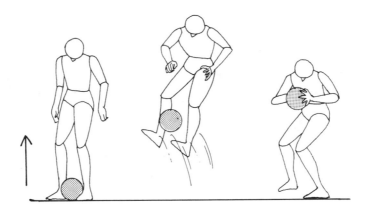

Front Toss. Stand with the ball held between your feet. Jump up with the ball, then toss it to yourself while in the air. *Ice skating, soccer, track & field.*

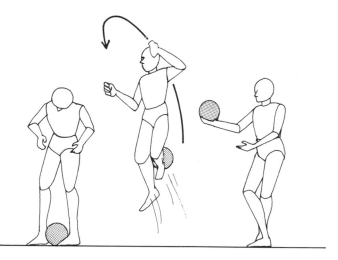

Heel Toss. Stand with the ball held between your heels. Jump up with the ball, toss the ball up and over your back and shoulders, and catch it in front of your body. This toss requires a quick snap of the hamstring muscles. *Soccer, baseball, track & field.*

Leg Toss

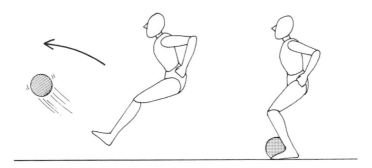

Leg Toss. Stand with the ball held between your feet. Jump up and pike in order to toss the ball out in front of your body. Be sure to jump upward before piking the hips. Try to throw the ball to waist level or over an object. *Track & field, soccer, gymnastics.*

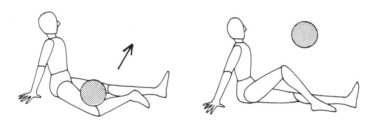

Knee Throw. Sit with one leg straight out on the floor and the other leg bent with the knee out to the side. Place the ball on top of the bent knee and use your hip and thigh to throw the ball across your other leg. *Soccer, golf, bowling.*

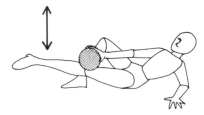

Inside Leg Lift. Lie on your side, and brace yourself on your elbow and lower arm. Place the ball on the inside of your knee that is against the floor and bend your other knee for balance. While holding onto the ball, lift your leg up six to eight inches and hold for a count of five. Do not allow your leg to rest on the floor until you complete the set. *Aerobics, cycling, gymnastics.*

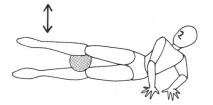

Double Leg Lift. Lie on your side and brace yourself with your hands. Hold the ball by squeezing it between your knees and lift both legs up off the floor four to six inches for a count of five. *Aerobics, ice skating, gymnastics.*

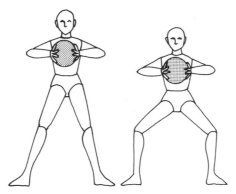

Dips. Stand with your feet a little more than shoulder width apart and feet turned slightly outward. While holding the ball in front of your chest with your elbows out to the side, lower your body by bending at your knees. *Aerobics, ice skating, gymnastics.*

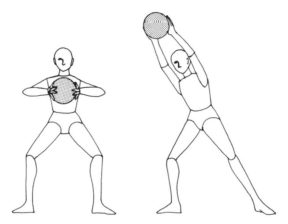

Dip Extension. Do a dip as described in the previous exercise, but instead of returning to your starting position, extend your arms and the ball above your head to one side of your body. When you extend to the right, your right leg will bend and your left leg will straighten out, and vice versa. Alternate between right and left extensions. *Volleyball, aerobics, ice skating.*

Split Squat

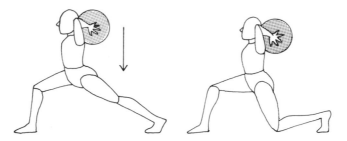

Split Squat. Stand with one foot out in front of your body. The forward leg should be bent and your rear leg should be straight. Hold the ball behind your neck and lower your body by bending the back knee toward the floor. Keep your upper body straight and perpendicular to the floor. Do not let your forward knee bend past 90 degrees or extend past your forward foot, and do not allow your rear knee to touch the floor. *Football, track & field, gymnastics.*

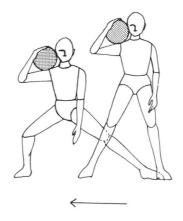

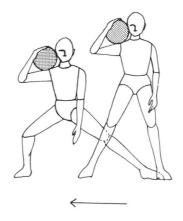

Side Lunge. Stand with your feet slightly more than shoulder width apart and hold the ball on one shoulder. Step out to your side with the foot that is under the ball and lower your body as far as possible. Push back to the starting position. *Ice skating, tennis, aerobics.*

Cradle Rocking

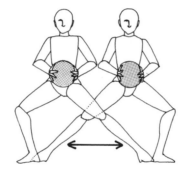

Cradle Rocking. Stand in a wide stance with your feet pointed outward. Hold the ball at waist level and rock from side-to-side over your feet without raising your body up and down. When you rock to the right, your right leg will bend and your left leg will straighten out, and vice versa. Keep your upper body straight and perpendicular to the floor. *Aerobics, tennis, racquetball.*

General Body Exercises with emphasis on Total Workout

General Body • Total Workout

In-Depth Jump with Chest Pass

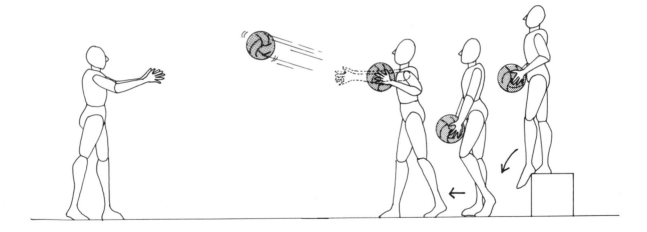

In-Depth Jump with Chest Pass. While holding the ball in front of yourself, start an in-depth jump by stepping off a box or other suitable elevated platform and land simultaneously on both feet. Instead of exploding upward and outward, take a quick step forward and do a chest pass in any direction. *Basketball, track & field, gymnastics.*

In-Depth Jump with Rebound Jump. While holding the ball in front of yourself, do an in-depth jump by stepping off a box or other suitable elevated platform and landing simultaneously on both feet. Explode upward and forward while extending your arms and ball upward. As you return to the floor, pull the ball down to your chest. Do a series of rebounds to increase the intensity of the exercise. *Basketball, volleyball, swimming.*

Catch and Pass in Different Direction

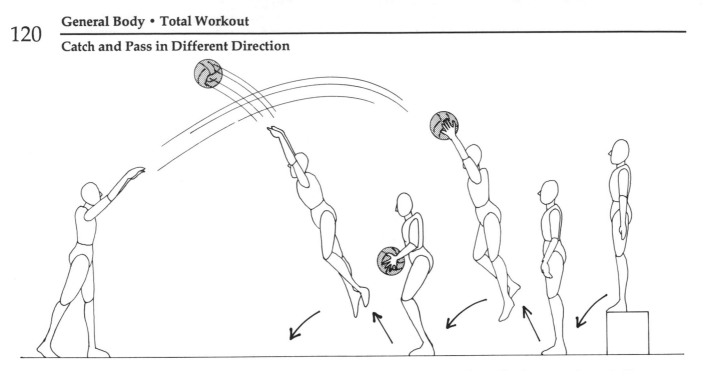

Catch and Pass in Different Direction. Do an in-depth jump by stepping off a box or other suitable elevated platform and landing simultaneously on both feet. Explode upward and forward, extend your arms, and catch a pass from your partner. Upon landing, explode upward again and pass the ball off in a different direction. *Basketball, volleyball, tennis.*

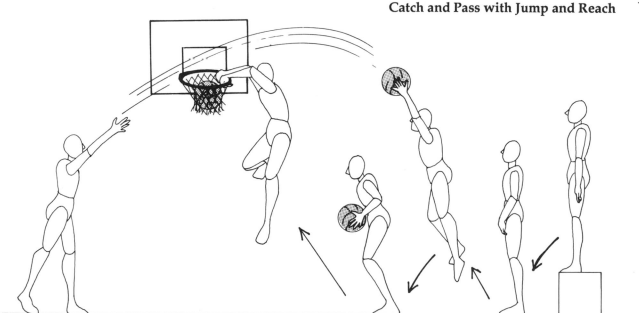

Catch and Pass with Jump and Reach. Do an in-depth jump by stepping off a box or other suitable elevated platform and landing simultaneously on both feet. Explode upward and forward, extend your arms, and catch a pass from your partner. Upon landing, explode upward again and reach for a high object such as a basketball goal. *Basketball, volleyball, track & field.*

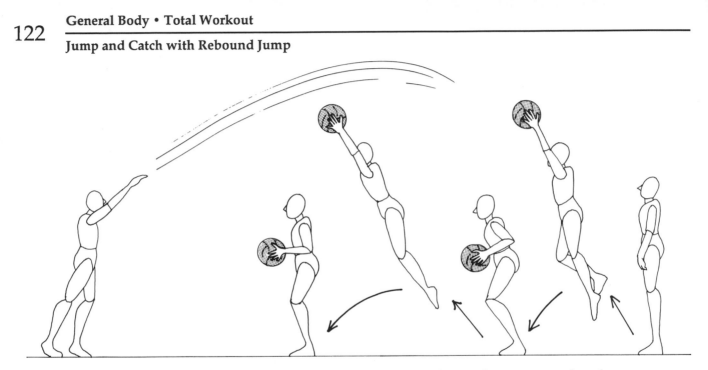

Jump and Catch with Rebound Jump. Jump upward and forward, extend your arms, and catch a pass from your partner. Upon landing, do a single rebound jump. For more exercise do a series of two to five rebound jumps. *Basketball, volleyball, track & field.*

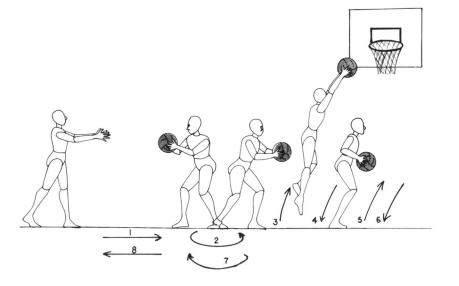

Big Man Drill. Stand with your back approximately three feet in front or to the side of the basket. Your partner starts the drill by tossing you the ball. Catch the ball, pivot, and jump to touch the ball against the rim. Immediately after landing, rebound and touch the rim with the ball a second time. Finally, pivot back toward your partner and toss the ball to him or her. *Basketball.*

Exercises
for
Wheelchair Athletes

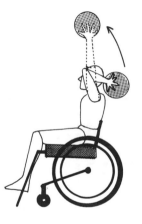

Tricep Press. Hold the ball behind your head with your elbows at ear level. Keeping your elbows steady and your back firmly pressed against the back of the chair, lift the ball up over your head to full arm extension. Then lower it back to the starting position. Do not allow your upper body to rock for momentum.

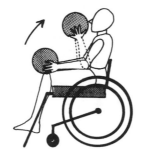

Bicep Curl. Hold the ball on top of your thighs with your elbows pressed into the front sides of your stomach area. Lift the ball upward to face level, then lower it back to the starting position. Do this exercise in a slow, smooth motion, and do not allow the ball to rest on your thighs until the set is completed.

Shoulder Flexion

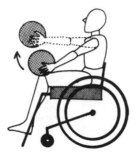

Shoulder Flexion. Hold the ball on top of your knees at full arm extension. Lift the ball upward to shoulder level while keeping your arms and back straight. Do not allow the ball to rest on your knees until the set is completed.

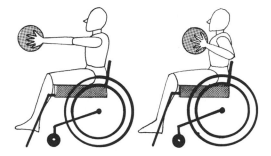

Chest Press. Hold the ball tightly in front of your chest with your elbows out to the sides. Press the ball forward to full arm extension, then draw it back to your chest. This exercise is to be done very forcefully and fast while keeping your upper body still.

Wrist Exercise

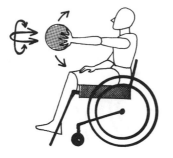

Wrist Exercise. Hold a small ball in front of your body with one hand at full arm extension. Your hand should be on the side of the ball. Move the ball in four different directions: up and down, left to right, clockwise, and counterclockwise.

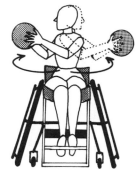

Twist. Sit as straight as possible while holding the ball in front of you with your arms bent. Twist your body at the waist from side to side. Twist your body as far as possible—go for distance in your turns, not speed.

Exercises for Wheelchair Athletes

Lateral Bend

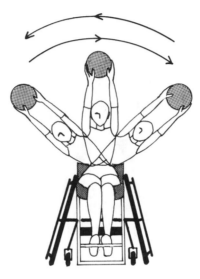

Lateral Bend. Hold the ball above your head at full arm extension. Bend your upper body at the waist from side to side while keeping the ball above your head. Do not allow your upper body to bend forward as each side bend is made.

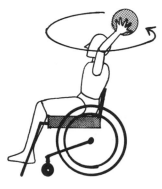

Seated Circles. Hold the ball at full arm extension above and as far behind your head as is comfortable. Move the ball in as large of circles as possible above your head while keeping your back against the chair. Do not allow your upper body to rock forward or sideways.

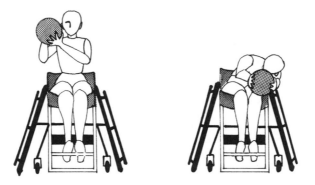

Diagonal Touches. While holding the ball on top of your right shoulder, bend forward until the ball touches your left knee. Lift your body and ball up to the starting position as one unit. Do not let the ball bounce off your knees, but keep the movement smooth and slow.

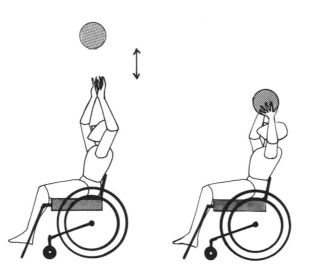

Overhead Toss. Lean back, look up, and hold the ball above your face. Press the ball upwards so that it leaves your hands, then catch it on its return. Immediately send the ball back up.

Exercises for Wheelchair Athletes

Over-The-Head Side Throw

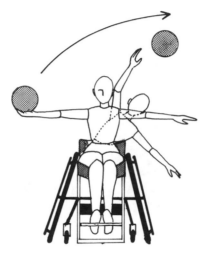

Over-The-Head Side Throw. Hold the ball in the palm of your hand and to your side at full arm extension. While keeping your arm stiff, use your upper body for momentum to throw the ball up and over your head to a catcher.

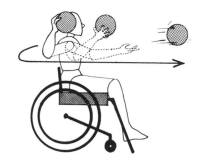

Side Throw. Hold the ball to the side of your head at ear level with your arm bent 90 degrees. As you throw the ball forward, your arm should move outward in a side arc. Your elbow should lead with your hand following, and your palm should be up when the throw is completed. This is the action used to throw a curve ball when pitching.

Exercises for Wheelchair Athletes

Chest Pass

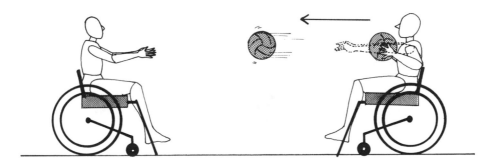

Chest Pass. You and your partner sit facing each other at a distance of six to ten feet. Hold the ball in front of your chest with your elbows out to the sides. Press the ball off your chest and pass it to your partner so that he or she can catch it at chest level. Move closer if the ball cannot be caught at chest level and keep the motion fluid.

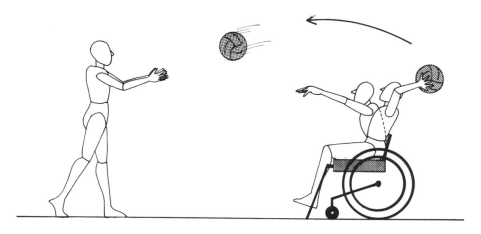

Overhead Throw. Hold the ball behind your head with arms extended. Throw the ball forcefully up and over your head to your partner. Your upper body should not fall forward as you throw the ball.

Exercises for Wheelchair Athletes

Backward Throw

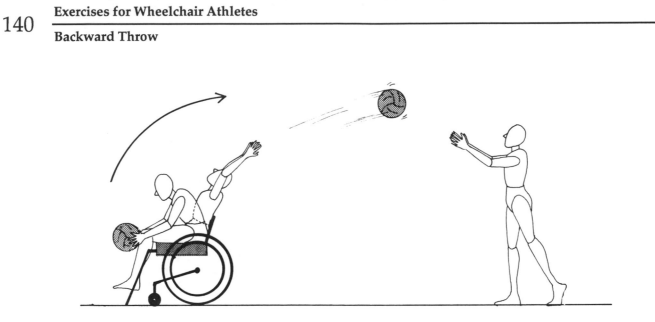

Backward Throw. Hold the ball at shin level at full arm extension. Throw the ball back, up, and over your head to your partner. Keep your arms extended and allow your body to go back against the chair, but keep your back straight.